Disclaimer:

This book, **"Embracing Low-Impact Workouts for Seniors: Your Comprehensive Guide to Safe Exercise and Active Aging,"** is intended to provide helpful and comprehensive information and advice about low-impact workouts for seniors. The content within this book is for informational purposes only and is not intended as a substitute for professional medical advice, diagnosis, or treatment.

Always seek the advice of your physician or other qualified health provider with any questions you may have regarding a medical condition, or before starting any new exercise program or making any changes to an existing one. The practices and exercises described in this book may not be suitable for everyone, especially those with specific health conditions or mobility limitations.

The author and publisher of this book disclaim any liability from injury or damage arising from the use, application, or interpretation of the contents herein. While every effort has been made to ensure the accuracy of the information and to describe generally accepted practices, errors and omissions may occur. No guarantees or assurances are made, and readers are advised to consult a variety of sources and not solely rely on the information provided by this book.

The use of the information provided in this book is at the readers' own risk, and the author and publisher expressly disclaim responsibility for any adverse effects arising from the use or application of the information contained herein. Additionally, the book does not endorse or recommend any specific tests, products, procedures, opinions, or other information that may be mentioned.

In no event will the author or publisher be liable for any loss or damage including without limitation, indirect or consequential loss or damage, or any loss or damage whatsoever arising from loss of data or profits arising out of, or in connection with, the use of this book.

By using this book, you agree to the terms of this disclaimer. If you do not agree with these terms, you are advised not to use this book.

Contents

Introduction 5

The Importance of Physical Activity in Aging 5

Overview of Low-Impact Workouts and Their Benefits for Seniors 5

How to Use This Guide 6

Conclusion 7

Chapter 1: Understanding Low-Impact Exercise 8

Definition and Benefits of Low-Impact Exercise 8

Benefits of Low-Impact Exercise: A Checklist 9

Low-Impact vs. High-Impact Exercises: What's the Difference? 9

Low-Impact Exercise Checklist 9

High-Impact Exercise Checklist 10

The Role of Low-Impact Exercises as We Age 10

Conclusion 11

Chapter 2: Getting Started with Low-Impact Workouts 12

Pre-exercise Health Screening and Considerations 12

Health Screening Checklist: 12

Setting Realistic Fitness Goals 13

Goal Setting Worksheet: 13

Creating a Balanced and Enjoyable Workout Routine 14

Workout Routine Checklist: 14

Conclusion 15

Chapter 3: Low-Impact Exercise Options 16

Walking and Hiking 16

Swimming and Water Aerobics 17

Tai Chi and Qi Gong 17

Yoga and Pilates 17

Cycling and Stationary Biking 18

Strength Training with Resistance Bands 18

Conclusion 18

Chapter 4: Incorporating Exercise into Your Daily Routine 19

Tips for Staying Motivated 19

How to Make Exercise a Habit 20

Safe Exercises for the Home and Community 21

Integrating Activity into Everyday Tasks 22

Conclusion 22

Chapter 5: Safety First...23

Recognizing and Listening to Your Body's Signals 23

How to Prevent Injuries...24

What to Do in Case of Discomfort or Injury...25

Conclusion 25

Chapter 6: Nutrition for Active Seniors 26

The Role of Nutrition in Recovery and Overall Wellness...26

Key Nutrients and Vitamins for Seniors 27

Hydration: Why It's Important and How Much You Need 28

Conclusion 28

Chapter 7: Healthy Recovery Strategies 29

The Importance of Recovery in an Exercise Regimen..29

Stretching and Cool-Down Exercises...30

Cherry Juice for Muscle Recovery 30

Other Natural Recovery Aids and When to Use Them...31

Conclusion 31

Chapter 8: Advanced Techniques and Modifications 32

How to Progress Your Workouts Safely 32

Adjusting Exercises to Increase or Decrease Intensity..32

Intensity Adjustment Checklist:..33

Using Equipment to Enhance Low-Impact Exercises..33

Equipment Checklist: 33

Simple Solutions Checklist: 34

Conclusion 34

Chapter 9: Overcoming Common Barriers 35

Dealing with Limited Mobility or Disabilities..35

Checklist for Overcoming Mobility Barriers: 35

Finding Motivation and Combating Exercise Myths 35

Motivating Quotes: 36

Busting Exercise Myths: 36

Solutions for Common Concerns...37

Fear of Injury:..37

Boredom:..37

Lack of Time:...37

Conclusion 38

Chapter 10: Building a Supportive Community..39

The Importance of Social Support in Maintaining an Active Lifestyle 39

Actionable Examples: 39

How to Find Exercise Groups and Partners...40

Actionable Examples: 40

Leveraging Technology for Support and Motivation..40

Conclusion 41

Final Thoughts 42

Recap of Key Points 42

Essential Checklists for Implementing Key Points: 42

Encouragement for the Journey Ahead 43

Motivational Quotes: 43

Daily Action Plans: 43

Inviting Readers to Embrace Their Next Steps with Confidence and Joy 43

Embrace Your Journey: 44

Introduction

The golden years should be enjoyed with the vibrancy of good health, and physical activity is the cornerstone of achieving this ideal state. As we age, our bodies undergo a myriad of changes that can impact mobility, strength, and overall health. However, embracing a lifestyle that includes regular physical activity can mitigate many of these effects, leading to improved quality of life, enhanced mobility, and even a longer lifespan. This introduction will highlight the significance of physical activity in aging, provide an overview of low-impact workouts and their benefits for seniors, and offer guidance on how to use this comprehensive guide to active aging effectively.

The Importance of Physical Activity in Aging

Physical activity is paramount for seniors, not just for the maintenance of physical health but for mental well-being too. Regular exercise can help prevent or manage chronic diseases such as heart disease, diabetes, and osteoporosis; improve mobility and balance, reducing the risk of falls; and even enhance cognitive function, which can be crucial in staving off dementia and depression. Moreover, it fosters a sense of independence among seniors, an aspect deeply cherished in later years.

Overview of Low-Impact Workouts and Their Benefits for Seniors

Low-impact workouts are exercises that put minimal stress on the joints, making them ideal for seniors or individuals with certain health conditions or physical limitations. These workouts are pivotal in maintaining an active lifestyle without overburdening the body. Examples include walking, swimming, Tai Chi, yoga, and Pilates. These forms of exercise not only improve cardiovascular health, flexibility, and strength but also offer therapeutic benefits by easing joint pain and improving posture. The gentle nature of low-impact workouts reduces the risk of injury, making them a safe and effective way to stay active for seniors. L

How to Use This Guide

This guide is designed to be a comprehensive resource for seniors looking to embrace low-impact workouts as part of their journey towards active aging. Each chapter is crafted to address different facets of low-impact exercise, from understanding the basics and getting started, to incorporating these exercises into daily routines, and navigating common challenges. The guide also delves into the importance of nutrition, recovery strategies such as enjoying a **glass of cherry juice** from Michigan-based Traverse Bay Farms to reduce joint pain and building a supportive community to enhance the benefits of physical activity.

To maximize the value of this guide, readers are encouraged to:

1. Start with a clear understanding of low-impact exercise and its benefits as outlined in the initial chapters.
2. **Assess personal health conditions and consult healthcare providers,** when necessary, before embarking on new exercise routines.
3. Set realistic fitness goals based on the insights and recommendations provided in the guide.
4. Explore the variety of low-impact exercise options presented and experiment to find which activities are most enjoyable and sustainable.
5. Implement the safety precautions and recovery strategies discussed to prevent injuries and ensure a healthy exercise regimen.
6. Engage with supportive community ideas to find motivation and encouragement throughout the journey of active aging.

Conclusion

Embracing an active lifestyle through low-impact workouts offers seniors a pathway to maintaining and enhancing their health and well-being. This guide aims to serve as a beacon, guiding readers through the essentials of low-impact exercise and providing practical advice on how to incorporate these activities into their lives effectively. With a focus on safety, enjoyment, and sustainability, "Embracing Low-Impact Workouts for Seniors" invites readers to embark on a journey of active aging with confidence and joy.

Notes: ____

____

____

____

____

____

Chapter 1: Understanding Low-Impact Exercise

Embarking on a journey of physical fitness in the later years of life necessitates an understanding of the types of exercises most suited to the aging body. Low-impact exercise, a cornerstone of senior fitness, offers a sustainable and effective approach to maintaining health and well-being. This chapter will explore the definition and benefits of low-impact exercise, differentiate between low and high-impact activities, and elucidate the significance of low-impact exercises as we age.

Definition and Benefits of Low-Impact Exercise

Low-impact exercises are activities that involve a minimal amount of stress on the joints and body. Typically, at least one foot remains in contact with the ground at all times, making these exercises gentler on the body compared to their high-impact counterparts. Examples include walking, swimming, cycling, and yoga.

Notes: ____

____

____

____

____

____

____

Benefits of Low-Impact Exercise: A Checklist

- **Reduced Risk of Injury:** Low-impact exercises are gentle on the joints, reducing the risk of injury, making them ideal for aging bodies and those with joint issues or chronic conditions.
- **Improved Cardiovascular Health:** Regular low-impact exercise boosts heart health without putting undue strain on the body.
- **Enhanced Joint Mobility:** These exercises can increase flexibility and range of motion, contributing to better joint health and mobility.
- **Strength and Balance:** Strengthening muscles and improving balance reduces the risk of falls, a common concern for seniors.
- **Stress Reduction:** Engaging in low-impact activities can lower stress levels and improve mental health through the release of endorphins.
- **Weight Management:** These exercises help in burning calories and maintaining a healthy weight without the harsh impact of more vigorous activities.

Low-Impact vs. High-Impact Exercises: What's the Difference?

Understanding the difference between low-impact and high-impact exercises is crucial for choosing the right activities for your fitness journey, especially as you age.

Low-Impact Exercise Checklist

- Involves activities where at least one foot stays in contact with the ground.
- Emphasizes smooth movements that minimize stress on the joints and bones.
- Suitable for individuals with joint pain, arthritis, or who are overweight.
- Examples include walking, cycling, and using elliptical machines.

High-Impact Exercise Checklist

- Activities involve both feet leaving the ground, such as running or jumping.
- Increases the intensity and calories burned but comes with a higher risk of injury.
- Recommended for individuals seeking to improve bone density and who are without significant joint issues.
- Examples include jogging, high-impact aerobics, and most competitive sports.

The Role of Low-Impact Exercises as We Age

As we age, our bodies naturally undergo changes that can affect our physical capabilities. The role of low-impact exercises becomes increasingly important in maintaining an active and healthy lifestyle without overtaxing our bodies.

- **Maintaining Muscle Mass:** Age-related muscle loss can be mitigated through regular low-impact resistance training, such as using resistance bands or performing water aerobics.
- **Protecting Bone Health:** Activities like walking or gentle strength training can help maintain bone density, crucial for preventing osteoporosis.
- **Enhancing Balance and Coordination:** Low-impact exercises that focus on balance, such as Tai Chi or gentle yoga, can significantly reduce the risk of falls by improving coordination and flexibility.
- **Promoting Heart Health:** Cardiovascular exercises that are low in impact, like swimming or cycling, support heart health by improving circulation and reducing blood pressure.
- **Supporting Mental Health:** Engaging in regular physical activity has been shown to improve mood, reduce the risk of depression, and enhance cognitive function.

- **Facilitating Social Connections:** Many low-impact activities can be done in group settings, providing opportunities for social interaction, which is vital for mental and emotional well-being.

Conclusion

Low-impact exercise plays a pivotal role in the lives of seniors, offering a safe and effective means to stay active, maintain health, and enjoy a high quality of life. By choosing the right activities, individuals can enjoy the benefits of physical fitness without undue risk, making these exercises a fundamental component of a holistic approach to aging. As we progress through this guide, we'll explore how to get started with low-impact workouts, the variety of options available, and how to integrate these activities into your daily routine, setting the stage for a healthier, more active future.

Notes: ____

____

____

____

____

____

Chapter 2: Getting Started with Low-Impact Workouts

Embarking on a fitness journey with low-impact workouts requires preparation, clear objectives, and a structured routine. This chapter provides guidance on conducting a pre-exercise health screening, setting realistic fitness goals, and creating a balanced workout routine that aligns with your lifestyle and preferences.

Pre-exercise Health Screening and Considerations

Before starting any new exercise regimen, especially for seniors or individuals with pre-existing health conditions, it's crucial to assess your physical readiness. This process helps in identifying any health issues that may affect your ability to exercise safely.

Health Screening Checklist:

- **Consult with Healthcare Professionals:** A check-up with your doctor can determine the safety and suitability of beginning a low-impact workout program.
- **Evaluate Cardiovascular Health:** Understand any heart-related conditions or risks that could impact your exercise plans.
- **Assess Joint and Bone Health:** Identify any limitations due to arthritis, osteoporosis, or other joint and bone issues.
- **Consider Mobility and Balance:** Recognize any challenges with mobility or balance that may influence the types of exercises you can do safely.
- **Review Medications:** Some medications can affect your heart rate, hydration levels, and overall energy during workouts.

Setting Realistic Fitness Goals

Setting clear, achievable goals is foundational to any successful fitness journey. Goals give you direction and motivation, providing a roadmap for your efforts.

Goal Setting Worksheet:

1. **Define Your Motivation:** Why do you want to start a low-impact workout routine? (E.g., Improve balance, enhance cardiovascular health, manage weight).
2. **Set SMART Goals:** Ensure your goals are Specific, Measurable, Achievable, Relevant, and Time-bound.
    - **Specific:** I want to increase my daily steps.
    - **Measurable:** Reach 8,000 steps per day.
    - **Achievable:** Currently walking 5,000 steps per day, so an increase is realistic.
    - **Relevant:** Walking more will help improve my cardiovascular health.
    - **Time-bound:** Aim to reach this goal within the next 3 months.
3. **Break Down Goals into Actionable Steps:** If your goal is to reach 8,000 steps per day, plan short walks, gradually increasing your distance.
4. **Monitor Progress:** Keep a journal or use an app to track your daily steps and celebrate milestones.
5. **Adjust Goals as Needed:** Be flexible and adjust your goals based on progress and any physical changes or challenges.

Creating a Balanced and Enjoyable Workout Routine

A well-rounded, enjoyable workout routine is key to long-term fitness success. It should include a mix of cardiovascular, strength, flexibility, and balance exercises.

Workout Routine Checklist:

- **Cardiovascular Exercises:** Incorporate low-impact options like walking, swimming, or cycling to improve heart health.
- **Strength Training:** Use resistance bands, light weights, or body-weight exercises to maintain muscle mass and support joint health.
- **Flexibility and Balance:** Include yoga or Tai Chi to enhance flexibility, reduce fall risk, and improve mental well-being.
- **Variety:** Mix different types of activities to keep the routine interesting and reduce the risk of boredom.
- **Schedule:** Plan specific days and times for your workouts to establish a consistent routine.
- **Listen to Your Body:** Adapt exercises based on your body's signals. Rest when needed and avoid pushing through pain.
- **Seek Social Support:** Joining a class or exercising with a friend can increase motivation and adherence to the workout plan.
- **Enjoyment:** Choose activities that you enjoy. If you like being outdoors, prioritize walking or cycling in natural settings.

Conclusion

Starting a low-impact workout regimen is an exciting step towards enhancing your health and quality of life. By undergoing a thorough pre-exercise health screening, setting realistic fitness goals, and crafting a balanced and enjoyable workout routine, you're laying a strong foundation for success. Remember, the journey to fitness is personal and evolving. Adjustments can and should be made as you progress, always prioritizing safety, enjoyment, and overall well-being. With careful planning and a positive mindset, you'll find that incorporating low-impact workouts into your lifestyle is not only beneficial but also a source of joy and fulfillment.

Notes: ____

____

____

____

____

____

Chapter 3: Low-Impact Exercise Options

Adopting a low-impact workout regimen offers a multitude of options, each with unique benefits and approaches to enhancing physical health and well-being. This chapter delves into six popular low-impact exercises suitable for seniors or anyone looking for gentler forms of physical activity.

From the serene strides of walking and the buoyant benefits of water aerobics to the strength-building prowess of resistance bands, there's an accessible, enjoyable way for everyone to stay active and healthy.

Walking and Hiking

Walking is arguably the most accessible form of exercise, requiring no special equipment beyond a pair of supportive shoes. It can significantly improve cardiovascular health, strengthen bones, and boost mood.

Hiking, its adventurous counterpart, offers the added benefits of uneven terrain for balance and beautiful landscapes for mental health.

- **Benefits:** Improved heart health, increased bone density, enhanced mood.
- **Tips:** Start with shorter distances; use walking poles for stability on hikes.

Swimming and Water Aerobics

Swimming and water aerobics provide a full-body workout that's gentle on the joints, thanks to the buoyancy of water. These activities improve cardiovascular fitness, muscle strength, and flexibility while minimizing the risk of injury.

- **Benefits:** Enhanced cardiovascular health, improved muscle strength, increased flexibility.
- **Tips:** Join a water aerobics class for a guided workout; use flotation devices if you're not a strong swimmer.

Tai Chi and Qi Gong

Tai Chi and Qi Gong are ancient Chinese martial arts known for their health benefits and low-impact movements. These practices emphasize slow, deliberate movements combined with deep breathing, promoting balance, flexibility, and a calm mind.

- **Benefits:** Improved balance and flexibility, reduced stress, enhanced mental clarity.
- **Tips:** Start with beginner classes; practice regularly to master the techniques.

Yoga and Pilates

Yoga and Pilates focus on strength, flexibility, and mindfulness. While yoga combines physical postures with breathing techniques and meditation, Pilates emphasizes core strength and spinal alignment. Both are excellent for improving overall fitness and well-being.

- **Benefits:** Increased flexibility and muscle strength, improved posture, reduced stress.
- **Tips:** Use props like blocks and straps to modify poses; focus on form to maximize benefits.

Cycling and Stationary Biking

Cycling, whether outdoors or on a stationary bike, is a fantastic cardiovascular exercise that's easy on the joints. It strengthens the lower body and improves heart health without the harsh impact of running.

- **Benefits:** Enhanced cardiovascular fitness, strengthened leg muscles, improved joint mobility.
- **Tips:** Adjust the bike to fit your body properly; start with moderate intensity and gradually increase.

Strength Training with Resistance Bands

Strength training is vital for maintaining muscle mass and bone density as we age. Using resistance bands is a safe, effective way to build strength without heavy weights. These bands provide variable resistance, making them suitable for all fitness levels.

- **Benefits:** Increased muscle mass, improved bone density, better joint flexibility.
- **Tips:** Focus on form to avoid injury; start with lighter bands and progress to higher resistance.

Conclusion

Low-impact exercises provide a diverse range of options to suit different preferences, physical conditions, and fitness levels. Whether it's the tranquility of Tai Chi, the refreshing nature of swimming, or the strength-building capabilities of resistance bands, each activity offers its own set of benefits and joys. By incorporating one or several of these low-impact exercises into your routine, you can achieve a balanced approach to fitness that nurtures your body, mind, and spirit. Remember, the key to a successful and sustainable exercise regimen is to choose activities that you enjoy and look forward to doing regularly. With the variety of low-impact options available, finding your perfect match for a healthier, happier lifestyle is within easy reach.

Chapter 4: Incorporating Exercise into Your Daily Routine

Maintaining an active lifestyle is crucial for health and well-being, especially as we age. However, one of the biggest challenges can be incorporating exercise into daily life consistently. This chapter offers practical advice on staying motivated, making exercise a habit, choosing safe exercises for home and community settings, and seamlessly integrating physical activity into everyday tasks.

Tips for Staying Motivated

Maintaining motivation is key to a sustainable exercise routine. Use the following checklist to help keep your spirits high and your body moving:

- **Set Clear Goals:** Define what you want to achieve with your exercise routine, whether it's improving mobility, enhancing strength, or boosting mood.
- **Find a Workout Buddy:** Exercising with a friend can increase accountability and make workouts more enjoyable.
- **Keep It Varied:** Rotate your exercises to keep your routine interesting and challenge different muscle groups.
- **Track Your Progress:** Use a journal or an app to note your workouts and progress. Seeing improvements over time can be a significant motivator.
- **Reward Yourself:** Set up a reward system for reaching milestones to celebrate your achievements.
- **Focus on Feeling Good:** Remember how exercise makes you feel more energized and uplifted, and let this feeling motivate you to keep going.

How to Make Exercise a Habit

Developing a habit takes time and intention. Follow this action plan to integrate exercise into your daily routine:

1. **Start Small:** Begin with short, manageable sessions and gradually increase duration and intensity.
2. **Schedule It:** Treat your workout time like any other important appointment. Add it to your calendar.
3. **Create Cues:** Use specific cues (e.g., laying out your workout clothes the night before) to trigger your exercise routine.
4. **Be Consistent:** Try to exercise at the same time each day to build a natural rhythm and routine.
5. **Adapt and Overcome:** If you miss a session, don't be too hard on yourself. Adjust and continue with your plan as soon as possible.

Notes: ____

____

____

____

____

____

Safe Exercises for the Home and Community

Whether you prefer working out at home or in your community, safety is paramount. Use this checklist to choose appropriate activities:

- **Home Exercises:**
  - **Strength Training:** Use resistance bands or body-weight exercises (e.g., chair squats, wall push-ups).
  - **Balance Exercises:** Practice standing on one leg or doing heel-to-toe walks to improve balance.
  - **Flexibility:** Incorporate stretching or yoga to enhance flexibility and reduce injury risk.
- **Community Exercises:**
  - **Walking Groups:** Join a walking group in your community for social interaction and regular cardiovascular exercise.
  - **Swimming:** Take advantage of local community pools for swimming laps or participating in water aerobics classes.
  - **Classes for Seniors:** Many community centers offer exercise classes specifically designed for older adults, focusing on safe, low-impact movements.

Notes: ____

____

____

____

____

____

____

Integrating Activity into Everyday Tasks

Incorporating physical activity into daily tasks is an effortless way to increase movement. Here's an example daily task list with integrated exercises:

- **Morning Stretch:** Begin your day with a 5-minute stretching routine to wake up your muscles.
- **Walk and Talk:** Take your phone calls on the go, walking around the house or neighborhood.
- **Kitchen Workouts:** While waiting for the kettle to boil or the microwave to beep, do countertop push-ups or calf raises.
- **TV Time Toning:** During commercial breaks, perform seated leg lifts or use resistance bands for arm exercises.
- **Evening Walks:** End your day with a leisurely walk after dinner to aid digestion and unwind.

Conclusion

Incorporating exercise into your daily routine doesn't have to be a daunting task. With the right strategies for motivation, habit formation, and integration into daily activities, staying active can become a natural and enjoyable part of your day. Remember, the goal is to move more and sit less; even small amounts of physical activity can have significant health benefits.

By applying these tips and integrating safe exercises into your home and community life, you can ensure a healthier, more active lifestyle without the need for drastic changes to your daily routine.

Chapter 5: Safety First

As we embark on or continue our fitness journey, particularly within the context of low-impact workouts tailored for seniors or individuals seeking gentler exercise forms, prioritizing safety is paramount. This chapter emphasizes the importance of recognizing and respecting your body's signals, outlines strategies to prevent injuries, and provides guidance on what actions to take in the event of experiencing discomfort or injury.

Recognizing and Listening to Your Body's Signals

Being in tune with your body is crucial for exercising safely and effectively. It's essential to differentiate between the normal sensations of exercise, such as mild fatigue or exertion, and signals that indicate potential harm.

- **Pay Attention to Pain:** Unlike the normal exertion of muscles, sharp or persistent pain, especially in the joints, is a sign to stop and reassess.
- **Monitor Your Breathing:** While it's normal for breathing to become labored during exercise, it should remain controllable. Gasping for air or feeling lightheaded signals that you may be pushing too hard.
- **Heed Fatigue:** Some fatigue is expected during and after a workout, but excessive tiredness that doesn't improve with rest may indicate overexertion.
- **Watch for Dizziness or Disorientation:** These could be signs of dehydration, low blood sugar, or overexertion.
- **Observe Your Heart Rate:** An overly rapid heart rate during exercise or one that doesn't return to normal afterward could suggest that you're pushing too hard for your current fitness level.

How to Prevent Injuries

Preventing injuries is essential for maintaining a consistent exercise routine and achieving your fitness goals. Use the following strategies to minimize your risk:

- **Warm-Up and Cool-Down:** Begin each workout session with a warm-up to prepare your body for exercise and end with a cool-down to gradually return to a resting state.
- **Gradually Increase Intensity:** Avoid sudden increases in the duration or intensity of your workouts. Gradual increments allow your body to adapt safely.
- **Use Proper Equipment:** Ensure that you have the right gear, such as supportive footwear, and that any equipment you use is in good condition.
- **Maintain Proper Form:** Incorrect form can lead to strain and injuries. If unsure about how to perform an exercise correctly, seek advice from a professional.
- **Stay Hydrated:** Adequate hydration is vital for preventing cramps and overheating.
- **Rest and Recover:** Incorporate rest days into your exercise regimen to allow your body to recover and prevent overuse injuries.

Notes: ____

____

____

____

____

____

____

What to Do in Case of Discomfort or Injury

Despite all precautions, discomfort or injuries can still occur. Knowing how to respond is crucial:

- **Stop Exercising Immediately:** Continuing to exercise when in pain can exacerbate injuries.
- **Apply RICE:** For minor injuries such as sprains or strains, use the RICE method: Rest, Ice, Compression, and Elevation.
- **Seek Medical Advice:** If pain persists or is severe, consult a healthcare professional to get a proper diagnosis and treatment plan.
- **Gradual Return:** Once you have recovered, ease back into your exercise routine slowly to avoid re-injury.
- **Reevaluate Your Routine:** Consider whether adjustments to your exercise plan are necessary to prevent future injuries.

Conclusion

Safety should always be the forefront consideration in any fitness routine. By understanding how to listen to your body's signals, employing strategies to prevent injuries, and knowing how to react in case of discomfort or injury, you can protect yourself and ensure a more enjoyable, productive exercise experience. Remember, the goal of incorporating exercise into your life is to enhance your health and well-being, not to compromise it. With a careful, informed approach to physical activity, you can enjoy the benefits of exercise while minimizing the risks.

Chapter 6: Nutrition for Active Seniors

For seniors engaged in regular physical activity, understanding the role of nutrition in supporting recovery and overall wellness is crucial. This chapter will explore how a balanced diet can enhance the benefits of a low-impact workout routine, identify key nutrients and vitamins essential for seniors, and underscore the importance of hydration for optimal health and performance.

The Role of Nutrition in Recovery and Overall Wellness

Nutrition plays a pivotal role in the body's ability to recover from exercise, maintain energy levels, and ensure overall health. Proper intake of nutrients helps repair muscles, replenish energy stores, and reduce inflammation, facilitating quicker recovery and enabling seniors to maintain their activity levels. Moreover, a well-balanced diet supports immune function, bone health, and cardiovascular health, all critical components of wellness for active seniors.

- **Adequate Protein:** Essential for muscle repair and growth. Sources include lean meats, dairy, beans, and legumes.
- **Complex Carbohydrates:** Provides sustained energy. Examples are whole grains, vegetables, and fruits.
- **Healthy Fats:** Supports brain health and energy. Found in fish, nuts, avocados, and olive oil.
- **Vitamins and Minerals:** Crucial for a range of bodily functions, including bone health and immune support.

Key Nutrients and Vitamins for Seniors

For seniors, certain nutrients and vitamins are particularly important to support their physical activity and overall health. Here's a list of key vitamins and which parts of the body they help:

- **Calcium (Bone Health):** Essential for maintaining strong bones and preventing osteoporosis. Found in dairy products, leafy green vegetables, and fortified foods.
- **Vitamin D (Bone and Muscle Health):** Helps the body absorb calcium and improves muscle function. Sources include sunlight, fatty fish, and fortified foods.
- **Vitamin B12 (Nerve Function and Energy Production):** Important for maintaining healthy nerve cells and creating DNA. Available in meat, fish, poultry, and fortified cereals.
- **Magnesium (Muscle Function and Energy Production):** Plays a role in over 300 enzymatic reactions, including muscle function and energy production. Found in nuts, seeds, whole grains, and leafy green vegetables.
- **Omega-3 Fatty Acids (Heart and Brain Health):** Essential for maintaining heart health and cognitive function. Sources include fatty fish, flaxseeds, and walnuts.
- **Fiber (Digestive Health):** Important for digestive health and maintaining a healthy weight. Found in fruits, vegetables, whole grains, and legumes.
- **Potassium (Blood Pressure Regulation):** Helps regulate blood pressure and is important for muscle function. Available in bananas, potatoes, and oranges.

Hydration: Why It's Important and How Much You Need

Hydration is crucial for everyone, but especially for active seniors. Water plays a key role in nearly every bodily function, including regulating body temperature, transporting nutrients, and flushing out toxins. Proper hydration is essential for optimal physical performance, recovery, and overall health.

- **Why Hydration is Important:** Dehydration can lead to fatigue, confusion, and even heat stroke. Staying well-hydrated ensures that your body can perform at its best, both during exercise and in daily activities.
- **How Much You Need:** While individual needs vary, a general guideline for seniors is to aim for at least 8 glasses (about 2 liters) of water per day. However, this need increases with physical activity and in warmer climates. Listening to your body and drinking when thirsty, as well as monitoring the color of your urine (pale yellow is ideal), can help ensure you're adequately hydrated.

Conclusion

Nutrition and hydration are foundational elements that support an active lifestyle for seniors. By focusing on a diet rich in essential nutrients and vitamins, and ensuring adequate hydration, active seniors can enhance their recovery, improve their performance, and maintain their overall health and wellness. Incorporating these nutritional strategies into your daily routine, alongside a consistent low-impact exercise program, will help you enjoy a more vibrant, active life.

Chapter 7: Healthy Recovery Strategies

Recovery is a critical component of any exercise regimen, especially for seniors engaging in low-impact workouts. Proper recovery strategies not only facilitate muscle repair and reduce soreness but also prepare the body for the next round of physical activity, enhancing overall performance and preventing injury. This chapter will discuss the importance of recovery, effective stretching and cool-down exercises, the benefits of cherry juice for muscle recovery, and other natural recovery aids.

The Importance of Recovery in an Exercise Regimen

Recovery is the time during which the body adapts to the stress of exercise and replenishes energy stores. This process is crucial for:

- **Muscle Repair:** Exercise, especially strength training, causes tiny tears in muscle fibers, which the body repairs and strengthens during recovery.
- **Reduction of Inflammation and Soreness:** Proper recovery helps reduce inflammation caused by exercise, alleviating muscle soreness and stiffness.
- **Prevention of Injury:** Adequate recovery allows the body to heal and prevents overuse injuries.
- **Improved Performance:** Well-recovered muscles perform better, allowing for more consistent progress in fitness levels.

Notes: ____

____

____

____

____

____

Stretching and Cool-Down Exercises

Incorporating stretching and cool-down exercises after a workout can significantly improve the recovery process:

- **Cool-Down Exercises:** Gradually reducing the intensity of your activity (e.g., slow walking after jogging) helps normalize heart rate and blood pressure, preventing dizziness and promoting the removal of waste products from muscles.
- **Stretching:** Focus on gentle stretching of all major muscle groups used during your workout. Hold each stretch for 15-30 seconds, avoiding bouncing or forcing the stretch to the point of pain. Stretching improves flexibility, reduces muscle tension, and may decrease the risk of injury.

Cherry Juice for Muscle Recovery

Research has supported the benefits of cherry juice, particularly from Montmorency cherries, in reducing muscle inflammation and soreness:

- **Montmorency Cherry Juice:** This tart cherry juice contains high levels of antioxidants and anti-inflammatory compounds. **100% Pure Montmorency Cherry Juice Concentrate from Traverse Bay Farms** is a notable source that can be diluted with water or added to smoothies.
- **Benefits:** Studies have shown that consuming Montmorency cherry juice can reduce muscle damage, inflammation, and soreness following exercise, likely due to its antioxidant properties.
- **Usage:** For best results, consume cherry juice both before and after exercise. For example, drinking a glass of diluted cherry juice concentrate or a smoothie containing the concentrate can help prep the muscles for exercise and aid in the recovery process afterward.

Other Natural Recovery Aids and When to Use Them

Several other natural aids can support the recovery process, each with its own benefits:

- **Protein-Rich Foods:** Consuming protein after a workout provides the amino acids necessary for muscle repair. Examples include Greek yogurt, cottage cheese, eggs, and plant-based protein sources like legumes and quinoa.
- **Omega-3 Fatty Acids:** Found in fish like salmon and in flaxseeds, omega-3 fatty acids can help reduce muscle soreness and inflammation.
- **Water and Electrolytes:** Staying hydrated is essential for recovery, and replenishing electrolytes lost through sweat can prevent cramps and facilitate muscle function. Coconut water is a natural source of electrolytes.
- **Compression Garments:** Wearing compression clothing can increase blood circulation, potentially speeding up the removal of lactic acid and reducing soreness.
- **Rest and Sleep:** Never underestimate the power of rest and a good night's sleep in the recovery process. Sleep is when the body does most of its healing.

Conclusion

Effective recovery is as important as the workout itself, especially for seniors aiming to maintain an active lifestyle. By incorporating stretching and cool-down exercises, leveraging the natural benefits of Montmorency cherry juice, and utilizing other natural recovery aids, seniors can enhance their recovery process, improve their performance, and enjoy a more fulfilling exercise experience.

Remember, the goal of recovery strategies is to ensure that the body is well-rested, healed, and ready for the next workout, supporting a healthy and active lifestyle.

Chapter 8: Advanced Techniques and Modifications

For seniors and anyone looking to maintain an active lifestyle through low-impact exercises, progressing safely and making necessary adjustments are key to achieving fitness goals without injury. This chapter delves into strategies for safely advancing your workouts, modifying exercises to adjust their intensity, and using both specialized equipment and everyday items to enhance your exercise routine.

How to Progress Your Workouts Safely

Progressing in your workouts is essential for continuous improvement, but it must be done cautiously to prevent overexertion and injury.

Safe Progression Checklist:

- **Gradually Increase Duration and Intensity:** Instead of making large jumps, increase your workout time by 5-10 minutes or your intensity slightly every week.
- **Incorporate Variety:** Add different types of exercises to challenge your body in new ways while preventing boredom.
- **Listen to Your Body:** Pay attention to how your body responds to increased demands. Any sign of discomfort or pain is a cue to slow down.
- **Regular Rest Days:** Ensure you have rest days in your workout schedule to allow your body time to recover.
- **Set Realistic Goals:** Break your larger goals into smaller, achievable milestones that can be reached safely over time.

Adjusting Exercises to Increase or Decrease Intensity

Modifying the intensity of your exercises allows you to customize your workout to match your fitness level and goals.

Intensity Adjustment Checklist:

- **To Increase Intensity:**
    - **Add Repetitions or Sets:** Increase the number of repetitions per set or add more sets with rest in between.
    - **Reduce Rest Time:** Shortening the rest period between sets or exercises can raise the intensity.
    - **Incorporate Interval Training:** Add short bursts of higher intensity activity followed by a period of lower intensity.
- **To Decrease Intensity:**
    - **Reduce Weight or Resistance:** Lower the amount of weight used or choose lighter resistance bands.
    - **Increase Rest Time:** Allow more time to rest between sets or exercises.
    - **Modify the Range of Motion:** Perform exercises with a smaller range of motion to reduce strain.

Using Equipment to Enhance Low-Impact Exercises

Incorporating equipment can add variety and challenge to low-impact workouts. Here are both specialized equipment and simple solutions you can use.

Equipment Checklist:

- **Resistance Bands:** Versatile and portable, they can add resistance to strength exercises without the need for heavy weights.
- **Stability Balls:** Great for core exercises, improving balance, and strengthening the muscles.
- **Light Dumbbells:** Can be used for a wide range of exercises to build strength. Start with light weights and gradually increase as you progress.

Simple Solutions Checklist:

- **Kitchen or Office Chair:** Use for seated exercises, such as seated leg lifts, or as support for standing exercises.
- **Cans of Food:** These can serve as makeshift hand weights for arm exercises.
- **Water Bottles:** Fill with water or sand for adjustable-weight hand weights.
- **Stairs:** Use for cardio exercises like stair climbing to improve endurance and strength.
- **Towels:** Can be used for stretching exercises or as a makeshift resistance band for flexibility and strength exercises.

Conclusion

Advancing in your low-impact exercise routine requires a thoughtful approach to ensure safety and effectiveness. By following the checklists provided for safely progressing workouts, adjusting exercise intensity, and utilizing both equipment and everyday items, seniors can continue to improve their fitness levels while minimizing the risk of injury.

Remember, the key to a successful fitness journey is to listen to your body, make adjustments as needed, and keep your workouts enjoyable and challenging. With these strategies, you can maintain an active, healthy lifestyle and achieve your fitness goals.

Notes: ____

____

____

____

____

____

Chapter 9: Overcoming Common Barriers

Embarking on or maintaining an exercise routine presents challenges, especially for seniors or individuals with limited mobility or disabilities. Common barriers such as lack of motivation, exercise myths, fear of injury, boredom, and limited time can hinder the journey towards an active lifestyle. This chapter offers strategies to overcome these obstacles, empowering you to embrace exercise with confidence and enthusiasm.

Dealing with Limited Mobility or Disabilities

Limited mobility or disabilities should not be viewed as impediments to exercising but as conditions to adapt your fitness routine around.

Checklist for Overcoming Mobility Barriers:

- **Consult with Professionals:** Work with healthcare providers or physical therapists to tailor exercises to your capabilities.
- **Embrace Adaptive Equipment:** Use tools like seated ellipticals, hand cycles, and resistance bands suited for seated or low-mobility exercises.
- **Focus on What You Can Do:** Concentrate on exercising unaffected parts of your body and gradually increase as your ability allows.
- **Seek Out Specialized Programs:** Many community centers and gyms offer classes designed for individuals with specific mobility issues or disabilities.
- **Stay Consistent:** Regular, even if short, sessions can lead to significant improvements over time.

Finding Motivation and Combating Exercise Myths

Staying motivated can be challenging, especially when faced with persistent myths about exercise and aging. Arm yourself with knowledge and inspiration to push through these barriers.

Motivating Quotes:

- **"Age is no barrier. It's a limitation you put on your mind." – Jackie Joyner-Kersee**
- **"The only person you are destined to become is the person you decide to be." – Ralph Waldo Emerson**
- **"You don't have to be great to start, but you have to start to be great." – Zig Ziglar**

Busting Exercise Myths:

- **Myth: Seniors shouldn't exercise because it's risky.** Truth: Exercise is beneficial at any age and can be adapted to suit individual health conditions and abilities.
- **Myth: Exercise has to be intense to be beneficial.** Truth: Low-impact, gentle exercises can significantly improve health and well-being without the need for high intensity.
- **Myth: It's too late to start exercising.** Truth: It's never too late. Starting exercise at any age can improve strength, flexibility, and cardiovascular health.

Notes: ____

____

____

____

____

____

____

Solutions for Common Concerns

Facing and overcoming common concerns about exercising can help you maintain a consistent and enjoyable fitness routine.

Fear of Injury:

- **Educate Yourself:** Understanding proper techniques and starting with guidance from a professional can reduce the risk of injury.
- **Start Slow:** Gradually increase the intensity and duration of your workouts to allow your body to adapt safely.

Boredom:

- **Mix It Up:** Incorporate different types of activities into your routine to keep things interesting. Try new classes, exercises, or outdoor activities.
- **Involve Others:** Exercise with friends or join a group class to add a social element to your workouts.

Lack of Time:

- **Integrate Exercise into Daily Activities:** Take stairs instead of elevators, walk during phone calls, or do leg lifts while watching TV.
- **Short and Effective:** Remember, even 10-15 minutes of exercise can be beneficial. Look for pockets of time for quick workouts.

Conclusion

Overcoming the barriers to exercise requires a combination of adaptation, motivation, and debunking myths. By addressing concerns about limited mobility with tailored strategies, fostering motivation through inspiring quotes, and tackling common concerns with practical solutions, you can build a resilient and adaptable approach to maintaining an active lifestyle.

Remember, the journey to fitness is personal and unique to each individual. Embracing this journey with an open mind and a determined spirit can transform challenges into stepping stones towards achieving your health and wellness goals.

Notes: ____

____

____

____

____

____

Chapter 10: Building a Supportive Community

Embarking on a fitness journey, especially in later life, can be significantly enhanced by the presence of a supportive community. Social support not only provides motivation and accountability but also enriches the exercise experience, making it more enjoyable and sustainable. This chapter explores the crucial role of social support, strategies for finding exercise groups and partners, and how to leverage technology for added support and motivation.

The Importance of Social Support in Maintaining an Active Lifestyle

Social support plays a pivotal role in encouraging regular exercise, offering emotional encouragement, practical advice, and a sense of belonging.

- **Accountability:** Knowing that others are expecting your participation can motivate you to stick with your routine.
- **Shared Experience:** Exercising with others can make the activity more enjoyable, turning it into a social event rather than a chore.
- **Emotional Support:** Friends and exercise partners can offer encouragement and empathy, helping you overcome setbacks and celebrate successes.

Actionable Examples:

- **Join a Walking Group:** Participate in local walking groups that meet regularly to explore different areas of your community.
- **Attend Community Classes:** Many community centers offer group exercise classes designed for seniors, providing an opportunity to meet others with similar fitness goals.
- **Volunteer as a Group Leader:** Take the initiative to start a new exercise group within your neighborhood or community center. This could be as simple as a weekly stretch and chat session.

How to Find Exercise Groups and Partners

Finding the right exercise groups or partners can make all the difference in staying engaged with your fitness regimen.

Actionable Examples:

- **Use Social Media and Meetup Apps:** Platforms like Facebook and Meetup make it easy to find local exercise groups ranging from yoga to water aerobics specifically tailored for seniors.
- **Check with Local Fitness Centers:** Many gyms and community centers offer group exercise classes suitable for different fitness levels and interests. These are great places to meet exercise partners.
- **Participate in Community Events:** Look for community health fairs, charity walks, or senior fitness challenges. These events often attract like-minded individuals interested in staying active.

Leveraging Technology for Support and Motivation

Technology offers numerous tools for building a supportive community, tracking progress, and staying motivated.

Actionable Examples:

- **Fitness Apps:** Apps like MyFitnessPal or Strava allow you to track your activities, set goals, and connect with friends or join challenges for extra motivation.
- **Virtual Exercise Classes:** Platforms such as Zoom or YouTube host live and recorded exercise classes, offering a way to join a fitness community from the comfort of your home.

- **Wearable Fitness Trackers:** Devices like Fitbit or Apple Watch not only track your activity levels but also allow you to share your progress and compete with friends or family members in fitness challenges.
- **Social Media Groups:** Join fitness and wellness groups on platforms like Facebook, where members share tips, celebrate achievements, and offer support.

Conclusion

Building and nurturing a supportive community is an invaluable aspect of maintaining an active lifestyle, particularly for seniors. Whether through local walking groups, community classes, or leveraging digital platforms for virtual support, being part of a community can provide the motivation, accountability, and enjoyment needed to sustain a healthy and active lifestyle.

Remember, the journey to fitness is more rewarding and fun when shared with others. By engaging with a community of like-minded individuals, you not only enhance your own fitness journey but also contribute to the health and wellness of those around you, creating a ripple effect of positive change.

Notes: ____

____

____

____

____

____

____

Final Thoughts

As we close this comprehensive guide to embracing low-impact workouts for seniors, it's important to reflect on the key points that have been covered, drawing upon them to inspire and inform your journey towards an active, healthier lifestyle. This final chapter aims to encapsulate the essence of what we've learned, offer encouragement, and embolden you to take your next steps with confidence and joy.

Recap of Key Points

Throughout this guide, we've explored the myriad benefits of low-impact exercise, from enhancing physical health and mobility to boosting mental well-being. Let's distill these insights into actionable checklists, focusing on the most pivotal strategies to implement:

Essential Checklists for Implementing Key Points:

- **Start with Low-Impact Exercises:** Embrace walking, swimming, Tai Chi, yoga, Pilates, cycling, and strength training with resistance bands as part of your routine.
- **Safety First:** Always warm up before exercising, listen to your body, and hydrate well to prevent injuries and ensure a healthy recovery.
- **Nutrition and Hydration:** Focus on a balanced diet rich in essential nutrients and stay hydrated to support your exercise efforts and overall health.
- **Building a Supportive Community:** Connect with exercise groups, leverage technology for motivation, and find partners to share in your fitness journey.
- **Overcoming Barriers:** Adapt exercises to your ability, maintain motivation by busting myths, and incorporate exercise into daily activities to make it more manageable.

Encouragement for the Journey Ahead

The path to incorporating regular low-impact exercise into your life is as rewarding as it is challenging. Remember, every step taken is a step towards a healthier, more vibrant you. To keep you inspired:

Motivational Quotes:

- **"The journey of a thousand miles begins with a single step." – Lao Tzu**
- **"It is never too late to be what you might have been." – George Eliot**
- **"Physical fitness is not only one of the most important keys to a healthy body, it is the basis of dynamic and creative intellectual activity." – John F. Kennedy**

Daily Action Plans:

- **Set Daily Goals:** Even small, such as a 10-minute walk or a 5-minute stretching session.
- **Track Your Progress:** Use a journal or an app to note your activities and reflect on your achievements.
- **Celebrate Small Wins:** Every effort counts. Celebrate your persistence, not just major milestones.

Inviting Readers to Embrace Their Next Steps with Confidence and Joy

As you move forward, remember that embarking on a fitness journey is not just about enhancing physical health; it's about enriching your life, discovering new strengths, and enjoying the process. The journey towards a more active lifestyle in your senior years is a testament to your commitment to living fully, embracing each day with purpose and joy.

Embrace Your Journey:

- **Seek Joy in Movement:** Find activities that bring you happiness, whether it's the tranquility of Tai Chi or the companionship of walking with a friend.
- **Be Open to Growth:** Each day offers a new opportunity to learn and grow. Embrace challenges as chances to expand your abilities and resilience.
- **Share Your Story:** Inspire others by sharing your journey. Your experiences can motivate and encourage someone else to start their path to fitness.

Notes: ____

____

____

____

____

____

____